A Better Normal for Vaginal Dryness & Pain

Your Guide to Rediscovering Intimacy After Cancer

Tess Devèze

Published in Australia by ConnectAble Therapies Pty Ltd.

1510 Mills Road, Glen Forrest WA 6071, Australia
Copyright © 2023 Tess Devèze
All rights reserved.

Disclaimer: All care has been taken in the preparation of the information herein, but no responsibility can be accepted by the author for any damages resulting from the misinterpretation of this work. The content in this book shall not be used as an alternative to seeking professional and clinical advice.

For more information see www.connectabletherapies.com

ISBN: 978-0-6458244-6-9

CONTENTS

WHY I WROTE THIS BOOK

Hello! It's so wonderful to meet you. I'm Tess.

I thought before we get into the more 'intimate' details, I'd introduce myself and let you know what this book is about.

I was diagnosed with stage-three breast cancer in 2018, at the age of 36. At the time of my diagnosis, I'd been working in the sexuality sector for years. Over the years since my cancer diagnosis and endless treatments, only twice did a healthcare professional voluntarily bring up the topic of sexuality and only one booklet was recommended to me (which I had to go and find myself). The lack of information and support on this topic, both during and after treatments, was painfully noticeable.

Why aren't more resources available? Why are we so afraid to talk about this essential aspect of our lives?

First and foremost, I'm an occupational therapist (OT). What's an OT, I hear you ask? We are functional therapists and use specific approaches to promote independence and participation in 'occupations' which are any kind of meaningful life activity that occupies us. OT's help you do the day-to-day activities that you need and want to do, as best you can. This may include self-care tasks (shower, dressing, toileting), work related (vocational) tasks, social or community activities…and may also include sex!

My clinical experience is mostly in sexuality - during and after cancer treatments, brain-injury, neurological conditions, and those living with disability. Before moving solely to sexuality for people with cancer, disability and chronic illness, most of my work was in private and public hospitals across Australia, working in neurological rehabilitation. I love neuroscience, and most of my work is based on neurological concepts.

Other than having cancer and being a sexuality OT, I also work with sexuality and self-development pioneers 'Curious Creatures', based in Melbourne Australia. I've facilitated hundreds of workshops online and face to face for nearing a decade, teaching consent, better intimacy and communication skills. I've seen thousands of people's lives change through a deeper understanding of sexual intimacy.

Lastly, I've also studied somatic sexological bodywork at the Institute of Somatic Sexology. This training has given me a deeper understanding of how libido, pleasure, arousal and orgasmicity (cool word huh?) work on a physiological, neurological, and psychological level. These learnings form an essential part of this book.

Even with all my training, I've struggled. If you're struggling too, you're not alone (even if it doesn't get spoken about).

But it's not just about me. The contents of this book are also guided by you. I have a Facebook group 'Intimacy and Cancer' with thousands of people - all cancers, all genders - from over 49 countries, who share and support each other on this topic. My one-on-one clients have also been a huge source of learning, generously sharing their experiences.

It's been almost two years since releasing 'A Better Normal; Your Guide to Rediscovering Intimacy After Cancer', and the positive feedback I have personally been receiving from readers has been at times overwhelming. I am humbled, amazed and inspired by the impact and influence this book has had for those out there suffering.

But cancer treatments are *haaaaaard*, and so is reading! I wanted to know how I could reach more people, change more lives for the better through the contents in this book. In answer to that question, I've created the 'A Better Normal' mini-book *series*. It's a number of bite-sized treatment or side-effect specific mini-books, to help cancer patients and their loved ones maintain and grow connection, intimacy and sexuality. Each mini-book is created from the information in 'A Better Normal; Your Guide to Rediscovering Intimacy After Cancer', but broken down into simple, easy-to-read guides relative to your very specific needs, because often during and after treatments committing to a 300-page book feels overwhelming or is simply not possible.

Books in the 'A Better Normal' mini-book series are:

- 'A Better Normal for **Libido**; Your Guide to Rediscovering Intimacy After Cancer'

- 'A Better Normal for **Vaginal Dryness & Pain**; Your Guide to Rediscovering Intimacy After Cancer'

- 'A Better Normal for **Body Confidence**; Your Guide to Rediscovering Intimacy After Cancer'

- 'A Better Normal for **Chemotherapy**; Your Guide to Rediscovering Intimacy After Cancer'

- 'A Better Normal for **Hormone Therapy**; Your Guide to Rediscovering Intimacy After Cancer'

- 'A Better Normal for **Fatigue**; Your Guide to Rediscovering Intimacy After Cancer'
- 'A Better Normal for **Changes in Erection**; Your Guide to Rediscovering Intimacy After Cancer'
- 'A Better Normal for **Radiotherapy**; Your Guide to Rediscovering Intimacy After Cancer'
- 'A Better Normal for **Pain**; Your Guide to Rediscovering Intimacy After Cancer'

Or if you're after all of the above information (and more) in one place, the all-in-one book 'A Better Normal; Your Guide to Rediscovering Intimacy After Cancer' has everything you need.

If you end up with several mini-books in the series, that's pretty normal, as we don't have only one side-effect (geez, wouldn't that be nice!), and we can have the same side-effect from more than one treatment (like fatigue, or changes in libido). Cancer treatments impact us differently, which is why some books in this series are side-effect specific, and others treatment specific. So, you can pick and choose what is most relevant for you and where you're at. You'll also notice that some mini-books have repeated

5

information in them. That's because some information is essential and helpful, regardless of what your side-effect or treatment is (like the communication tips, or ways to gently reconnect with yourself or a partner).

The most important thing you can learn from this book is that you're not alone and you're not broken. There's nothing wrong with you if you're struggling. It's normal to find this situation tough. This isn't one-size-fits-all advice. All bodies are unique, every relationship is different, and everyone experiences relationships, connection, pleasure and desire in their own way. You're the expert on you! Just as cancer is different for everyone, so are the connections we have with ourselves and those around us.

Lastly, this book is for all human beings, regardless of gender, lifestyle, orientation, ability, ethnicity, age, or relationship dynamic. Although every person with cancer is unique, we have one thing in common: no matter who we are or what we are going through, we're all worthy of love and connection.

Now, let's get started on making your 'new normal', a 'better normal'.

1. KEY TERMS EXPLAINED

Sexuality vs sex

The word 'sexuality' is an umbrella term which yes includes the functional activity of sex, but also includes relationships, connections, affection, dating, pleasure and our overall well-being. Sexuality can be greatly affected due to cancer, but it doesn't necessarily have to stop altogether. As a sexuality educator and clinician, I know how important sexuality, connection and intimacy is to our quality of life, our resilience and coping. What could be more important!

'Sex' in this book refers to the act, or the activity you engage in with yourself and/others, and is one of the most diverse and most adaptable functional activities I can think of. Yet today, it's still one of the most under-addressed topics in clinical settings. This is something I aim to change.

I also want us all to be on the same page in how we see 'sex' itself which is more than just orgasms and genital play, it's so much more. During cancer treatments and other life-altering events, you might need to temporarily let go of traditional forms of touch/sex. We can become excited, aroused, release pleasure hormones in our body from so many different ways. There are erogenous zones all over our bodies such as our inner thighs, breasts, nipples, under the armpits, the neck, earlobes, feet and many more depending on your body. Orgasms, engorgement, ejaculation, becoming 'hard' or 'wet', these don't need to be your goal, but can also be experienced in more than one way. Pleasure, enjoyment, arousal, excitation and connection, that is where the fun can also be. Pleasure is pleasurable and our whole body can be pleasured!

Desire vs arousal

Desire (the wanting) I use interchangeably with libido. Desire/libido are the experience of *wanting* sex and pleasure. Desire has many words that can be used, such as lust, sex-drive, and essentially all refer to that *want* we have.

Arousal is the way our body responds when it's in pleasure, the changes in our body that show us we are in fact, enjoying and excited. Things like increased sensitivity, maybe we become wet, maybe we become hard, our heart rate increases, we breathe heavier and more.

Simply put, libido = wanting, and arousal = enjoying.

Treatments can affect our arousal as well as our libido, which I dive into in this book, but knowing the difference between these can be very helpful.

The magical word, intimacy

Disconnection from yourself and others is a common side-effect of cancer treatments for so many. You're not alone in this and here I introduce you to the magical word 'intimacy'. Imagine that you having sex or being intimate again with yourself, a date or a partner/s, is the goal or the prize. That prize is on the other side of a river, and to get to it, you need to build a bridge. How can you do that? Through intimacy, through touch and the other magical word *affection*.

I've heard many times from clients and people in my support group "we don't even touch each other anymore". Not only has sex gone, but so has the *intimacy*, and are we really going to want sex without that connection?

Intimacy and affection are small giants. Tiny little things that can mean the world, and build that bridge of connection. Things like hand-holding, a good-night kiss, a good morning hug, your arm around your partner in the kitchen, cuddling on the couch, touch for the sake of touch (not as a way to 'get somewhere'), massage swaps, maybe a cheeky butt-squeeze and grin, and the big one, WORDS OF LOVE.

When you want some touch or love? Here's a few ways to ask, without that pressure of it needing to lead to sex:

How to say it out loud.

- "Hey, I'd like to be closer to you, how about a cuddle?"
- "Can we snuggle together on the couch while watching this film?"
- "You up for some hand-holding while we walk to the shop?"
- "I'm loving you right now, thought I'd share."
- "You up for some underwear-on cuddling while we fall asleep? I miss connecting with you."
- "I'd love some touch/to touch your body, would you like a massage?"
- "I'm not wanting this to lead to sex, but some kisses and cuddles would be lovely if you're feeling like some connection?"
- "I'm checking you out right now, just wanted to share."

- "I'm running a bath to relax and wind-down from the day, would you like to join me for some down-time?"

Small giant steps towards that prize.

2.   CONNECTION

When people hear the word 'connection', some assume it means something to do with sex. Well, that is not necessarily always the case as there are so many different types of meaningful connection in our lives, which I'll discuss here.

Connection could be the sharing of intimacy through affection with another, or with yourself. It can make you warm, bring you closer to someone, provide feelings of value and being loved. A hug from a friend, a hand-hold from a family member, even a simple smile from a stranger. Connection, belonging, it all can have a positive impact on us.

Have you heard of the hormone oxytocin? It's referred to as the 'cuddle hormone'. Not only is this hormone released in the body during arousal, but softer, slower forms of touch, such as hand holding or cuddles (just to name a few) can also produce this pleasure hormone. This proves that you can still feel connected, even from the simplest forms of touch such as a hug or soft kiss on the cheek, and why intimacy is so important for our general wellbeing.

There will be relationships and connections in your life that become distant after a diagnosis and there are many reasons for this. Some relationships will struggle, some will fail, some simply might not understand how unwell you are and others might leave or pull away. I lost people during my treatments; people very close to me. I was not coping at all; I was struggling while trying to survive and put walls around me. It's sad, but not an uncommon story. Remember, one of the most difficult things you can experience during treatment is the challenge of putting yourself first. You're fighting for your life, you must. It's how you will manage to face each day. It's how you will survive. Know that other relationships can get stronger, deeper, more loving and connected, and you may even end up with stronger supports and connections around you than before.

Why connecting is essential

I want to share a 'light bulb' moment I had during chemotherapy, one that helped me change a lot about the way I connected to those around me.

I was 4 months into chemotherapy and had just switched to having chemo weekly. It was a sweltering 38-

degree Australian summer night and I walked out of a poetry reading with a friend, to go home. While walking, he hooked his arm through mine, as a sign of affection and connection. When his arm linked through mine, I noticed that I jumped at the touch. Noticing my reaction and how much I had been startled at the contact, it dawned on me. How long had it been since I had been touched in a way that was not medical, hurried and detached? Three weeks? Maybe four? I was so used to the non-intimate hands of nurses, oncologists, surgeons etc. who were not aggressive, but let's say, purposefully unaffectionate in their touch. It was a shock to receive this wonderful soft, intimate connection of an arm slipping through mine. I realised I had become an object of analysis and procedure, and was no longer one of affection. It was shocking to me and it also saddened me.

That was the moment I realised I was losing connection, that was the moment I saw I was becoming detached and I needed to be more vocal. The people around me were being respectful and careful not to touch me, due to how unwell I was. I loved everyone's respectful approach and care towards me as I was very, very sick. I'm grateful for their care, but I realised they also needed guidance from me, to know what was okay and when.

Realising the only touch I had been receiving was medical, which I would switch off to and detach myself from, was one of those 'ahaaa' moments. I had realised how disconnected I had become to my body and that I needed to make the first move and communicate. So, I beg you, educate those around you. Tell your friends they can hold your hand, your family members can put their arm around you, a partner or lover can snuggle with you on the couch. Be their guide for your connection.

3. COMMUNICATING'S HARD, BUT IMPORTANT

Please don't be down on yourself if you're struggling (whether you're a partner or the person diagnosed). Things are hard, things are different. It's okay, there are workarounds (which I'll get into soon). Ignore external pressures and expectations and focus on yourself and each other. Not only do our bodies and lives change from cancer, so do our roles. From partner to patient, lover to carer, friend to carer etc. You can get through it, together.

Silence is the enemy and can be common when we're finding things difficult. Fear and uncertainty are prevalent during treatments and we can withdraw from each other intentionally or unintentionally. It makes sense that we don't talk about the thing that's hard to talk about!

Fear of dating, meeting new people, of hurting a partner, not knowing how their/your new body works or not wanting to cause pain can all be reasons someone withdraws. Plus, your partner/loved one has seen you go through one of the hardest things of your life, be more unwell than ever, it's scary stuff.

For reasons above and more, not knowing how to

interact and pulling away is common.

For the people with the diagnosis, understanding what is happening in our body and communicating that? That can feel impossible. Either way, humans have not evolved to read minds, so you'll need to break the silence and share what's happening. So often, the concerns we have in our minds seem a lot bigger when they stay in our minds. Talking is key.

And while we're at it, please don't compare yourself to anyone else or any other relationships. It's the fastest way to unhappiness at any level and that includes comparing yourself to yourself, the 'pre-cancer you'. I call myself 'Tess BC' (BC = before cancer) when I'm in that loop. I often think of my pre-cancer body and mind, how I used to have less pain, more energy, body parts that used to be there, how I could remember things and focus on tasks, so you're not alone in this. I constantly remind myself, comparisons to others or the way things used to be won't change anything. It's such an easy pattern to fall into. I'm sorry to be so blunt as it's hard not to think about what has changed and how things used to be, but please try to think ahead. Cancer is different for everyone and every relationship is different.

There are millions of us fighting cancer, with suffering sexuality. It can be scary, but you don't have to do this alone.

Who to ask and how to ask

Communication with your loved ones isn't the only thing that's essential, but also communication with your treating team. Knowing who to ask about sexuality, positioning, care & *safety* is something most of us don't know.

Here's a general summary.

Gynaecologists work with people who have a vulva and/or vagina. Urologists work with those who have a penis. Gastroenterologists and colorectal surgeons work with the digestive system including bowel cancers. Haematologists work with blood and lymphatic cancers. You will also have medical professionals relative to your treatments such as a radiation oncologist for radiotherapy treatments, an endocrinologist for hormone treatments and the effects they have on our bodies and sexuality, and your oncologist who oversees your treatments. You will have a surgical team relative to the type of procedure you will be having. Psychiatrists are who to speak with regarding mental health and medications, including which medications have which impacts on your sexuality.

All of these people plus your nurses, your doctor or GP (general practitioner if you're in Australia) are all trained to answer your questions.

There are also people like me (OTs) who focus on sexuality, there's pelvic floor physiotherapists and OTs, there are sexologists and sex counsellors as well. You will need to ask; you will need to be your own advocate for your sexuality. But don't worry, if they're not sure how to best answer your question, they will find someone who is. Your care is their priority.

I hear you saying "sure Tess, it's easy to tell us to ask medical professionals questions, but *how* do you ask the questions?" The first step (asking) is the hardest…. But you can do it, I've got your back!

How to say it out loud.

- "How will this treatment affect me sexually?"

- "What are the precautions I need to take regarding sexual activities during this treatment?"

- "Do I need to avoid sex or do specific things safety-wise? If so, when and for how long?"

- "What do I and my partner/s need to know or do regarding intimate activities?"

- "I'd like to ask a few questions about sex and intimacy during my treatment. Is there a more private space we could go to?"

- "Is there someone I can speak with, who can answer questions about sex during and after treatment?"

- "We/I would like to discuss intimacy during/after treatment. Can we organise a time? And with who?"

- "I'm experiencing some changes with my (vagina/vulva/genitals). Who is the best person to speak to?"

- "How will this treatment affect me/us intimately?"

- "How long after surgery should we wait until it's okay to have sex again? And are there any positions or movements we should avoid?"

- "I'm not sure how to ask this, but I have some questions of a more private nature, who can I speak with about that?"

- "What are the precautions I need to take regarding sexual activities during chemo?"

- "I'm experiencing some genital discomfort, who can I speak with about that?"

If a healthcare professional isn't sure or cannot answer your question?

- "Thanks for letting me know, can you please ask someone who might be able to answer?"
- "Okay, can you please tell me who I can ask?"

4.   OUR POOR VAJOOTZ (VAGINAL PAIN & ATROPHY)

For people with a vulva, genital pain is *very* common from treatments. To just quickly explain some words if 'vulva' is new to you; the vagina is the internal portion of the genitals. It refers to the internal canal, where things like tampons, cups, speculums, toys, fingers and penises can go into. Vulva is the word for the parts of the genitals on the outside; including the labia, vaginal entrance (the vaginal introitus), mons pubis (pubic bone), clitoral hood, shaft and head etc. 'Atrophy' is a medical word for tissues thinning, breaking down or getting weaker. From various treatments (chemo, radio, endocrine, surgeries impacting or removing sexual organs), vulva and vaginal tissues can get 'roughed up' so to speak and cause discomfort and pain.

Words like 'sandpaper', 'burning' or 'glass-shards' are used to describe the pain felt during internal play. And for people like me, pain felt all day every day during even the simplest of things like walking, sitting or simply wearing underwear. Atrophy and pain can interfere with quality of life, with daily function, cause social and romantic isolation, and isn't something to be ignored.

Why you should have caution when you hear 'use it or lose it' regarding vaginal pain

I honestly can't believe how many people are told by healthcare providers "use it or lose it" in regards to painful penetrative sex. Please, *please*, have caution. The "use it or lose it" motto is a statement for people that work in neuroscience. It's used to describe the process of neuroplasticity in regards to neurological rehabilitation, say after brain or spinal cord injury, NOT musculoskeletal issues. It certainly doesn't apply for pain. Being told you should have painful sex to heal the painful sex is like someone telling you that walking on your broken leg will help it heal.

I think what is happening here is that clinicians know that blood-flow is the number one way to heal tissues, and for the vaginal canal, getting aroused is a way to get blood to that area. Clinicians also understand that the vaginal canal can maintain its elasticity with 'use'. What clinicians seem to be leaving out of this conversation, is the understanding that many of us do not or cannot have vaginal penetration, and that intentionally causing ourselves more pain can be traumatic to ourselves and to our partners. I have supported people who have forced themselves to have painful and unwanted penetrative sexual experiences because they thought it was their only option (quoting this badly-used-motto to me), which has resulted in more damage physically and also psychologically. Speaking from a consent and trauma perspective, this is not okay.

There are endless ways to have sex, to get aroused, to get blood flow to your pelvis, and strengthen the internal muscles, all without having to be penetrated and potentially cause you more harm. Pain is your body's alarm system telling you something is wrong. And, if you're forcing yourself to have painful sex, your brain is going to start to associate sex as something that is bad/negative/painful/a source of anxiety/stressful and you will WANT IT LESS. It's the ultimate libido killer (if you're experiencing drops or changes in libido, take a look at the mini-book 'A Better Normal for Libido' for ways to recover it).

Are you still on treatments? If you're still on treatments like endocrine treatments, your atrophy won't completely recover as you're still taking the thing that causes it. But you can totally help improve it a *lot*, which I will cover shortly. Also, if you're on endocrine treatments/had internal radiation, the vaginal entrance or canal can shrink a bit, which can be another source of pain. As mentioned in the mini-book 'A Better Normal for Radiotherapy', you can use dilators, fingers or toys to maintain canal size and shape, if you wish.

Dilators are objects of varying sizes that are inserted into the vaginal canal regularly, to maintain canal shape, size and function. Use varies from using internal creams and dilators for a few weeks, to using them over years or even permanently. I know some who include dilator use each morning in their shower routine, others who experience pain need to be slow and careful, so need to carve considerable time (and energy) out of their day. This can be an extremely difficult thing to manage and endure, and can hold a lot of trauma. Please have discussions with your endocrinologist, radiation therapist and/or gynaecologist regarding your particular situation and vulvovaginal concerns, as dilators are not always the answer. These are only to be used if recommended by a clinician, who has physically examined you and can prescribe the correct use, regime and ways to use them without causing further harm.

Regarding "use it or lose it", I've been speaking very strongly here, as I see so many people hurting themselves and having negative sexual experiences because they think it's their only option, or that they *should* just force it and grit their teeth through the pain. This isn't helping anyone. So, here are some other options and ways we can lessen vaginal pain and maintain function, without doing more damage.

1. Stop.

As mentioned, please avoid penetrative forms of sex while it hurts, as you'll only make it worse. Avoiding penetrative sex doesn't mean avoiding sex all together, you can still have a lot of pleasure and sex in other ways, which I share throughout this book. Remember, pro-tip: Sex should never, ever hurt. If we put up with pain and have sex we don't enjoy, we will start associating the act of sex as something that is not enjoyable and, in turn, *want it less*.

2. Chat.

Have someone physically take a look at your vulva and/or vagina for an accurate diagnosis. Someone who knows your treatments, your body, your cancer and what is safe for you. There are other possibilities than just atrophy which can cause vulvovaginal pain, such as vulva eczema, inflamed Bartholin's glands at the vaginal entrance, vaginismus, vulvodynia or lichen sclerosis. Seeing a professional for an accurate diagnosis is vital for your recovery and well-being. If you're not satisfied with the recommendations of who you see, you can always seek another medical professional.

3. Moisturise.

Just like we moistures our hands when they're dry and cracked, you'll need to moisturise your vagina. And regularly. There are internal moisturisers of all brands and types, shop around and find what suits you. How often you need to use moisturisers will vary depending on the severity of your dryness/atrophy, your type of cancer and your day-to-day functionality, so contacting your doctor, oncologist or gynaecologist is important. Please ask your doctor before purchasing one and speak with the pharmacist when you're there, about any medications/treatments you're on. There may be ingredients that will cause a reaction to your internal tissues, the only way to know if something could benefit you, is to consult with your treating team.

Some vaginal moisturisers have hormones in them such as oestrogen or testosterone, and there are creams that mimic a steroid ('prasterone') our body naturally produces in our adrenal glands. If you have a hormone receptive cancer, this may be risky. If you don't have a hormone receptive cancer, internal moisturisers containing hormones may be a life-saver for you. Again, consult your doctor. If you need a hormone free internal moisturiser, look for anything that contains hyaluronic acid. It's a slick substance we produce naturally in our bodies to keep our synovial joints moving smoothly and it's *great* for our vulvovaginal tissues.

I use internal moisturisers at night before going to bed. I literally put the moisturiser in while I'm lying-in bed about to try and sleep. I suggest this because moisturisers can leave discharge, and when we're walking about during the day, gravity can cause the moisturiser to drip out. Letting it be absorbed overnight while we're lying down is great. If you need to use them during the day or in the morning, wearing period underwear is a nice way to absorb any discharge and still be comfortable.

4. Lube.

The #1 way to know if you likely do have atrophy, is if you feel discomfort and pain during vaginal penetrative sex even when you're using lube.

Why would you still experience pain if you're using

lube? If you have vaginal atrophy, lubricants aren't going to help, because the problem isn't friction/needing things to be slippery (which is the sole purpose of lubes), the problem is the health of your internal tissues. Lubes don't fix pain, they prevent it. This is where we need to use internal moisturisers as described above.

I recommend using lubricants even when you aren't experiencing discomfort, because lubes make good things great and reduce friction. But if you're new to buying them, the choices can be overwhelming, so here's some tips.

The human body is an extremely complex organism and is designed to self-heal, so when your internal tissues are dehydrated and damaged, your body sucks up water like a sponge. That's why, when it comes to vaginal atrophy, water-based lubes are *not* the best. If we don't constantly top-up while playing, we're at risk of doing more damage, as we get dry inside quickly (as we've absorbed the water) and that dryness causes rubbing and friction. Plus, some water-based lubes once absorbed leave a residue inside us, and this can actually cause *more* friction than if you weren't using a water-based lubricant at all.

When in doubt, use a silicone-based lube. These are super slick and don't get absorbed into our bodies nearly as fast. Silicone lubricants aren't great to use on silicone toys (as they can break down the toy over time), but that's okay, just pop a latex condom over the toy and you're good to go.

Oil-based lubes are also great like organic coconut oil, as they also last longer. If this language is new to you, I'll cover the types of lubricants that are out there in more detail, shortly in the section titled 'lube is life'.

There is also a wax-based product called 'olive & bee' which is fantastic for anyone experiencing discomfort internally, and can be used as a lubricant *and* an internal moisturiser. The natural wax and olive oil has healing properties and feels great on sore tissues.

Remember, lubes don't help tissues heal, they only prevent doing tissue damage through reducing friction. So, using a moisturiser regularly as well as using lubricants every time you play internally is key.

5. Massage
Vulvovaginal massage is the number one way to help heal vaginal tissues while maintaining pleasure. Gentle, slow massage once or twice a week gets blood-flow to your tissues promoting healing, but is also a way to regain sensitivity through (you guessed it) neuroplasticity. If this is

all sounding very new and you wouldn't know where to start, I teach vulva massage (on yourself or with a partner) in the 'Vulva Pleasure Masterclass' described at the end of this book in the 'resources' section. It's not nearly as scary as it sounds. Remember, massage feels great and with a slow approach (which I guide you through), it can be wonderful for healing dryness and pain.

6. Pleasure.

Yup, I want you to self-pleasure. Not internally though as it might cause you more pain and increase tissue damage. I mean you or a partner offer pleasure externally. Clitoral stimulation, anal stimulation and other erogenous zones. Arousal gets blood to the deep tissues inside your pelvis and around your genitals, which promotes healing.

Having difficulties getting aroused on/after your treatments or meds? Use a vibrator on your clitoris and/or anus (more on that later in the 'it's toy-time' section). They work a treat and remember, you can have sex, pleasure and orgasms without having to be penetrated, especially while it hurts.

If you're feeling numb or desensitised on your clitoris and/or vulva, chat to your doctor about trying a 'scream

cream' which is a prescription cream locally put onto your clitoral and vulva area 30 minutes before intimacy. It enhances blood-flow and sensitivity. If you are someone with genital herpes, let your doctor/pharmacist know, so they can make up a formula that reduces the risk of causing a breakout.

7. Exercise.

Light exercise such as walking or yoga puts your pelvis in motion and gets blood circulating. It may seem strange, but this can have wonderful benefits for strengthening your pelvic muscles and healing vaginal tissues, as it gets the blood flowing. Try 15-20 minutes per day of brisk walking, but remember anything is better than nothing, so even 5-10 minutes a day will help. If walking isn't your thing, I highly recommend a free online yoga teacher on YouTube. Her channel is called 'Yoga With Adriene' and she has so many fantastic classes and programs, to suit anyone and everyone.

Anything that gets your pelvis moving and the blood flowing is a win, so find what works for you.

8. Bathe.

Just as walking is great to get blood-flowing, so is a warm

soak in the bath. It relaxes the muscles, the joints and gets blood to the internal tissues (noticing a theme here?). If you don't have a bath, pop a *warm* (not hot) wheat-pack or *warm*-water bottle between your legs if it feels soothing. It will still get the blood flowing and help heal.

If you're using dilators or other objects to insert into your vaginal canal, getting your body warm and relaxed beforehand can help make the experience more comfortable.

9. Oil.

Not only can we have internal atrophy, but also external. The vulva tissues on the outside of your body, like your labia and around the vaginal entrance can be sore. Applying some organic coconut oil, or even internal moisturisers on the outside of your genitals after the shower can help replenish the tissues and ease pain. Some people also use organic coconut oil internally as a substitute for an internal moisturiser. Find what's right for you.

10. Underwear.

Breathable, natural and comfortable underwear is important. I switched to 100% natural bamboo underwear as cotton was too painful for me. My vulvovaginal atrophy and pain were so bad I got to the point where I could barely walk, putting my entire life on hold. We're all different, so try a few things out. When I found the right brand for me, I nearly cried from the relief from the pain when I put them on.

And speaking of underwear, with vaginal and vulva pain, menstruation for many is a very stressful and painful experience. Sanitary pads, tampons, cups and other insertables can be painful to use and for me, caused of a *lot* of anxiety. There are however, brands of 'period underwear' with inbuilt absorbent padding and are machine washable. As someone who was sceptical, but gave them a go as tampons were excruciating for me to use, I was pleasantly surprised by how well they work and how comfortable they are. Each country has its own brand, so I won't recommend one specifically, but these are an incredible option to manage menstruation, while avoiding the pain and stress of having to insert anything.

11. Allied Health.

Not only do you have your oncologist, gynaecologist and other specialists on your side, but there are also pelvic floor physiotherapists, osteopaths and occupational therapists who specialise in this. You don't have to do this alone! All countries have their own unique medical and referral systems, but you won't know what's out there and who you can access unless you ask.

A note of caution: There are creams that have numbing agents which can be inserted into the vaginal canal to numb pain when being penetrated, and as incredible as this may sound, I need to ensure you're careful. Just like lubricants, numbing creams don't heal pain. They simply temporarily numb an area of the body, reducing sensation and pain. So, if you're using a numbing cream, say for penetrative sex while you have internal atrophy, you won't feel pain (your body's warning system that it's being hurt), and may do more harm. Some people notice they are in even more pain once the cream wears off, as they have further damaged their tissues. Numbing creams can be used, but it's essential you only use them if advised by your gynaecologist or medical professional who has examined you. You don't want to cause more damage, more pain and in turn, create more stress around sex.

Touching on laser treatments.

In several countries around the world, there are vaginal treatments which use lasers to 'ease' atrophy and its side-effects. I'm yet to read the results of any studies on these treatments, so have no evidence-based perspective on this. I do know some countries have banned this 'treatment' as the lasers were not designed to treat atrophy (hence the lack of evidence that it's safe and appropriate to use), plus the people operating them are often not medically trained. Some countries however, have clinics up and running and have staff with clinical training. It seems to be a 'treatment' with no industry standard yet, so have caution.

I've heard mixed results from people. By mixed I mean it has been wonderful for some and not at all for others. Please don't book a session without chatting with your gynaecologist or oncologist first. They're not cheap and may not be suitable or safe for you. If you've had internal vaginal radiation therapy, internal lasers may not be an option for you, so it's vital for your safety that you speak to a gynaecologist.

5. SIMPLE IDEAS FOR CONNECTING

Something we often do, especially in intimacy, is develop patterns. So often I support people whose intimacy and sex, revolves around vaginal penetration. And when that's not possible due to pain, people can get intimately distant from themselves and each other, as they're not sure what else their sex can look like.

In this section I give you some ways you can have a date-night with someone (or yourself!) which allows you to have fun, connect with yourself, feel good in yourself and feel good with others. The ultimate ideas to keep your sexuality and pleasure alive and present, if vaginal penetration is your normal form of sex, and isn't possible right now.

The activities I've listed and described are ones I've taught, read about and love to do - and are my top picks for you to try yourself. It's not an exhaustive list, but will give you a start (i.e., trust yourself and you can decide what works for you). Not all will appeal to you, that is fine. They are varied enough so that hopefully there's something for everyone that seems appropriate to try.

Remember, these can be done to the level that is right for you, with the person that is right for you. These can be done with a close friend, your carer, by yourself, partners and even family members!

Q&A

I am obsessed with this verbal game and full credit to Roger Butler from Curious Creatures who created it. It's so useful and fun to play if you're in a position where you want to communicate with someone, but it's hard to bring up an awkward topic or start a conversation. It's also great to play any time anywhere, and I love it in social or private settings. It's so simple yet an incredible way to deeply communicate and connect with strangers, loved ones, friends and everyone else. This game is a godsend for us feeling emotionally connected and safe, and these are the drivers for our intimacy. During many of my treatments, I struggled (and still do) to keep up with conversations that involved more than two people as the brain-fog/cancer-brain had my attention span so low. I also struggled at times to have conversations about how I was feeling and where I was at. I often played Q&A as a way to be able to listen to one person at a time, and still have valuable, connective conversations with the people around me. I also play it one-on-one to have meaningful conversations with a partner or friend, while communicating was/is so difficult. Simply put, Q&A makes good conversation great, and when you're struggling, it's a life-saver.

How it works.

Someone asks a question, any question, such as: How was your day? How are you feeling in your body? What do you love about your partner right now? What is your relationship to your sex? Do you like cake more than ice-cream? Anything.

The person sitting to the left of the person who asked the question, answers it first. When they are finished, it goes to the next person to the left, finishing with the person that asked it. If you're in pairs, the person who asked the question, answers it last.

There are a few extra rules:

- Every answer is perfect.
- Every question is perfect.
- No interrupting someone's answer, wait until they have told you they are finished answering, before

sharing your thoughts.

- You can 'pass' on a question (or make something up!).

- You can call 'Tangent' or 'Time' by making a 'T' symbol with your hands. This indicates that someone may be off on a tangent or taking too much time to answer. We always say "thank you" for a 'T'.

- The person who asks the question, always answers it last.

It may seem strange, having a verbal Q&A game in a book about intimacy around vaginal pain and dryness, but there's a theme here. Cancer interrupts life, which includes relationships. Medications, fatigue, nausea, stress, it all interferes and open communication for some can seem too hard. Try this game, try it a few times, it was and still is, a 'go-to' for me, when I want to connect.

Where? You can play it anywhere. Try it in the bath, the couch, at dinner, in the car, a BBQ, your fortnightly or monthly relationship check-in, or a few rounds at the end of the week to see how you're going. It's a beautiful time to be honest, because the rules are that you can't be interrupted and every answer is perfect.

This is also your saving grace if conversations are hard, paying attention is tricky and keeping up with multiple people talking at once. If you let people know what you need and where you're at, they will most likely help you out. I noticed social chatter was a way for people to let me know that 'everything was fine'. But it wasn't, I couldn't concentrate, I couldn't follow the conversation, I quickly forgot what people were saying and I got super stressed. As soon as I mentioned I needed conversation to slow down, that's exactly what happened. Remember, you will need to let people know what you need, and they will be grateful for the guidance. Q&A is a brilliant way to have social structure, and still offer wonderful connections with everyone present.

Little, lovely treats

Sit down and write a list of 5 - 10 things that are small and easy to do, that make you feel special or connected to yourself. Little, lovely treats. If you have a close friend or loved one, get them to do the same, write a list of little lovely things they enjoy. This could be a foot massage, a bath, a favourite wine, a nice cheese with salami and a childhood film (my personal favourite), moisturising each other's hands/backs/necks/chests, looking at photos together, a blindfolded touch experience, a game of loving Q&A (just described in this section) or dancing to your favourite music.

So, when a time comes, when you're feeling like you would like to connect, be intimate, share affection and don't know what to do? Get the list out and see what you're/you're all in the mood for.

All of these small treats should ideally be things that can be done in your home or very close to where you're staying, and don't take a lot of energy. You want your energy to be spent on connecting and enjoying yourself and others' company, not setting up or travelling to a location.

These 'small treats' lists are your go-to. When you're stuck in your head or having a bad day, get the list out. Soak your feet and moisturise them, do yoga, have a self-pleasure session or pleasure a partner, eat an entire pizza when those taste-buds are back online or get your favourite film and a pot of your favourite tea. The point is that you want an easy way to feel special involving yourself, and possibly those close to you. Simple, sensual, special treats that connect you with yourself/others.

Warming and calming

This small yet intimate task can really let you relax, unwind and get connected. A gentle, beautiful way to connect with yourself or with someone else, is by enjoying a warm bath. Relaxing in a body of warm water (not too hot!) has so many positive effects on the body. Muscles relax, our nervous system down-regulates (relaxes), it can reduce stress, muscle tension eases, pain can lessen, blood circulation improves, the list goes on. Add a cup of tea, a glass of wine, something playing on a screen you can see or some quality Q&A (see earlier in this section) if you have a 'bath-buddy' with you.

The waterless bath

Baths not your thing or you don't have one? I have for you, the waterless bath experience. Pop your electric blanket on a nice low setting or warm up a heat pack on the couch and create a warm snuggly cocoon for yourself or for you and your pet, child, friend or lover. The intent is to create warmth, intimacy, safety and connection - baths are not essential for this, but feeling safe and snuggly is.

A royal bathing

Credit for this idea goes to my primary carer, who 'softens' the daily activities to connect and show love, and has also used this technique when caring for a friend while undergoing treatments for brain cancer (spoiler, they loved it!). Is your partner, lover, friend or carer helping you with your personal care? Such as dressing, washing or even simply helping you dry your feet after the shower? If this is the case, every once in a while, ask the person assisting with your care to take their time with it. Turn it into an almost worshipping, lovingly sensual dressing or bathing. Imagine the treatment someone might get in a luxury ancient Roman spa.

Slowly wash the feet, slowly caress and wash the back, take your time enjoying putting clothing on someone, let the materials softly brush over the skin. Attention and intention are drivers of pleasure and going slowly allows this to happen. Yes, we are often time poor and we go into 'automatic mode', however this is a lovely five-minute task which can be added into daily life quite easily and shows care, love and affection. This small activity acts as a reminder to each other, you're not in a clinical environment, you're not a nurse going through the rounds with a patient, you're caring for someone, someone you care about. Be soft, be gentle, be present. What a treat and what a connector. And it only needs to take an extra five minutes or so.

A simple good night kiss

Life is hectic and a cancer diagnosis doesn't lighten the load. Finances, appointments, family life, medications, symptoms and more, can fill up the days. The only time you may actually see a partner or lover is at the end of the day. If this is you, think about taking five minutes, when you're in bed together getting ready for sleep. Lie down facing each other and look into each other's eyes. Touch noses if you like, hold hands, intertwine feet, hold eye contact, share a good-night statement, breathe together or share a kiss on the lips. It's a time where you're both settling down and both in the same spot, it's a great time to use it to connect.

Don't go to bed at the same time as the person you live/share space with? That's okay, ask that you get 'tucked-in' or tuck your partner in. Get the blankets up to their chin, wish them good night, give them a kiss and a few words of love. It's just such a sweet thing. And if you don't share a house with your loved ones? Sweet, loving good night text messages mean the world!

Self-pleasure

Our entire bodies are capable of pleasure and giving yourself some time, some touch and love is a beautiful way to connect with yourself and get those happy chemicals flowing. During treatments you may be tired, stressed, sore, in pain or feeling flat. Whether you're single or partnered, a lovely way to calm and connect with yourself is to give your body, soft, loving touch. This can, but doesn't necessarily need to involve your genitals or you getting aroused. Our bodies are complicated things and treatments can make our body almost feel like a stranger, so getting to know it again can be wonderful.

Give yourself some time, show yourself you're special and set yourself a date. Be it once a fortnight, once a week, or whenever you feel slightly motivated. It's nice, the first few times if you try to leave genitals out of it, just to see what it's like to focus on your body in a different way. We don't give ourselves enough one-on-one time and this is most definitely the case for personal intimate touch. Be curious, explore, hug yourself, scratch, tap, softly touch the skin, find what your body is and isn't enjoying, what it does and doesn't enjoy at that moment. I'm a firm believer that offering ourselves self-pleasure and understanding our bodies is essential for us to be able to connect with others. Regardless if you're partnered or not, having some time with yourself is healthy, it's calming, and it's connecting.

Massage swaps

This may seem like a strange thing to recommend in regards to intimacy and pleasure, but hear me out. Touch, care, love and affection are all things many of us forget about during and after treatments. If you're unsure of what your body wants in an arousal, erotic sense, your immediate fallback plan can be massage. Having someone massage you, gives focus on physical, attentive touch without that pressure of it needing to lead to sex. It's pleasurable, it's intimate and gets you connected (and it feels so good!). Massage swaps can also act as an 'ice-breaker', if you're with a partner or on a date and it's been a while since you've touched each other (which is common). This is a lovely and accessible way to ease back into a physical and touch based dynamic without the pressure to 'perform' or 'be sexy'. If you're not partnered and want some touch, but aren't sure how? There are many very skilled professional massage therapists out there, even the 'pop-in' 10-minute massage parlours have amazing touch and anything that connects you to your body and feels good, is a win.

Another amazing benefit of doing massage swaps, is it's a way for a partner or lover to get used to touching your changed body. So often, I support partners through their fear and anxiety of hurting their partner by touching them. A simple massage can be a way to have your partner touch your body and even start to explore areas they are hesitant to touch (like surgery sites or scars). With a little encouragement, direction and permission from you, these fears and anxieties can be overcome, together.

An undressing ritual

When our body's change, how we see ourselves and also, the fear of being naked in front of another person (and ourselves) can greatly impact our intimacy and overall well-being. Changes in body confidence and self-esteem are one of the most common things I support people with (if you're struggling with body image and confidence, take a look at the mini-book 'A Better Normal for Body Confidence'). Undressing rituals are a method of removing clothing for yourself, or another, in a way that is gentle while allowing space for nervousness and shyness, while inviting acceptance and positive regard. You can do this solo by yourself in front of a mirror as a way to get used to your new body, or with a date or partners.

How it works.

There's a lot of scope for variety here so feel free to bend and change this to suit you, but here's the basics. Standing in front of a mirror or someone else, you choose one item of clothing at a time to take off, and as you remove it you make a personal statement. Something that is true, that is how you feel, but also as a way to process, release and move towards acceptance. It's a neat psychological trick and can be wonderful. If you're doing this with a partner, take turns, so after you remove an item of clothing and make a statement, they do the same. Then it's your turn again, and so on.

By statements I mean things like;

- As I remove my shoe, I let go of how hard I am on myself.
- As I take off my shirt, I let go of my self-consciousness.

- Removing my belt is me removing the restrictions of society's ridiculous beauty standards.

- As I remove my bra, I welcome in love and acceptance of my body.

- As I take off my scarf, I release my fear.

- By taking off my pants, I am freeing myself of anxiety.

- By removing my pink sparkly cowboy hat, I am letting go of my tiring day.

Or, if that form of statement doesn't feel right, you could try positive words as you remove clothing and show parts of your body:

- As I look at my arm, I notice the smooth skin I have.

- While looking into the mirror, I'm loving the freckles I have on my face.

- With my chest exposed I feel an appreciation for being alive.

- As I look at my genitals, I notice the awesome curls in my pubic hair.

- As I see my stomach, I see scars/marks of me living, and making it through.

- While looking at my lower back, I like the curve where it joins my bottom.

I have done this by myself in front of a mirror, with a long-term partner and also on a date. It was surprisingly effective on the date, as I was very self-conscious about my body and didn't know how to transition from clothed to well, not-clothed. We both took turns slowly removing an item of clothing, we looked into each-other's eyes, we were honest and it was magic. It helped me relax and it helped them understand how I was feeling and how I was struggling.

Go slow. If you're doing this alone in front of the mirror, it can be quite confronting. Don't feel like you need to fully undress, you may need to do this gradually over time. You could remove one additional item of clothing in the mirror to look at and love each time you do this, so it's nice and slow. I've done it several times alone, as a way to slowly look at myself and get used to my changed and abnormal body. I cried a lot, but it truly helped me with body acceptance and processing my grief for the body I used to have. Follow yourself, breathe and trust that you can stop if you need to. If you're with someone and you don't want to get naked, you can remove 'imaginary' items of clothing (like an orange feather boa, a sequin vest, rainbow suspenders etc.) or simply ask to stop. You could also do this with someone, where you take turns in removing an item of clothing off of the other person, while making positive statements about their body. Or maybe you choose the item of clothing on yourself to remove and your partner/date shares statements of love and appreciation of that particular body part. The best part of this activity is that there's room to change this to what feels right for you, at the pace that's right for you.

Chatty-massage

If you're liking the ideas in this book about communicating more about what you want and giving more feedback in intimacy and pleasure, but aren't really sure how to do that, this one's for you. 'Chatty massage' is very simple, and is the perfect way to get better at figuring out what you want or don't want, and also, how to ask for it. It's another great way to get sexy with someone without penetration, and is another excellent activity to do, if your partner is feeling a little hesitant to touch your body, because they're scared of hurting you.

How it works.

Easiest done in pairs, one of you is the 'masseuse', and the other receives the 'massage'. But there's a twist. The person lying down, the one receiving the 'massage' is actually directing the masseuse on what to do. Sounds easy right? Well, there's a little more to it.

The person who is receiving direction, the 'masseuse' is only able to do exactly that, receive and follow directions. They cannot take over the experience or offer what they *think* the person receiving might enjoy. They can only follow the directions given by the person lying down who is 'receiving' the massage. The most important part is, that if the masseuse/person following directions doesn't hear something along the lines of "keep going" or "I like this, continue please" or a new instruction, they must stop touching the person giving the directions all together by gently removing their hands and waiting for the next instruction.

Why does the person have to stop touching after 10 seconds of silence you ask? For the person who is receiving the directions, this is a lesson in being guided in touch, in taking feedback and more importantly, not making assumptions as to what the other person may want and 'winging it'. For the person receiving the massage/giving directions, it allows them to learn how to ask for what they'd like and how to communicate if they'd like something to stop, continue or to change. It's powerful stuff. It's also an incredible way for them to really explore their body and to learn what they do and don't like at the pace that's right for them.

Giving feedback and knowing how to receive it during intimacy is the thing that makes a good time, a delicious time. But we're not taught how to talk about sex or our bodies. We're definitely not taught how to explore our likes and dislikes in a safe and compassionate way. The world would be better if we were. Chatty massage (as simple as it seems) is your way to flex those communication muscles and learn so much about your and your partner's pleasure.

If you're not sure where to start, try doing it together sitting on the couch and just on the hand or shoulders to start with. Or have a clothes-on play together while you get used to how it works. You could even set a timer so you have 5 or 10 minutes each of giving and receiving while you're trying it out. You can start by exploring things like soft touch on your arms, maybe scratchy touch on your back, massage touch on your neck and thighs. Soft kisses on your lower back. Feel free to get creative as the person following directions is going to stop if you don't ask for it to keep going, or ask for something to change. This is the safety mechanism, so you both can feel free to relax and have a bit of fun with it.

You may be thinking that the more difficult role in this is the person who's lying down and giving the directions. Funnily enough, when I work with partners together and I teach them this activity it's the complete opposite. It's the person receiving directions and having to stop and withdraw touch after 10 seconds of silence that struggles the most! Due to this, I'm going to repeat the rule as it's surprisingly tough for people, but is so important. If the 'masseuse' doesn't hear a direction after 10 seconds, they must stop what they're doing, remove their hands and wait. This is what will help the person giving direction do exactly that, as they will *have* to give you direction when you stop. So much of our intimacy is guess-work and with the impacts of cancer treatments, clarity and communication could never be more important. Stopping the touch after a short amount of time is a way to help each other practice giving and receiving feedback and most importantly, tuning in to what you do and don't want at the time.

It will 100% feel clunky and awkward at first, just like everything else we try in life for the first time. Don't worry too much about it as this is play, and yes play can be clunky, but it can also be fun. Have a laugh and have another go. Communication is the number one sex move, and this activity is the perfect way to practise.

The two-minute game

Finally, we learn about the two-minute game! Life coach Harry Faddis created the 'three-minute game' and I was taught the 'two-minute game' from Roger Butler at Curious Creatures, and it's simply brilliant. This game is suitable for those experiencing treatment and their loved ones, is great when you have no idea how to connect with someone or where to start, is a wonderful way to gently get to know each other's bodies again and is perfect to be intimate around things like pain.

Here's the rules.

- Set a timer or an alarm on your phone for two minutes.
- Pick who goes first, then that person asks for something they would like for 2 minutes (some examples are listed shortly).

- If you all agree, start the timer and give the person whatever they asked for.
- When the timer goes off, completely stop what you're doing.
- Then it's the next person's turn to ask for something they would like for two minutes.
- If everyone agrees, start the timer and go.
- Once the timer goes off, again, stop what you're doing.
- And repeat.

That's it. Really, that is the game. So simple, yet so effective. You can play it for as long as you like - 10 minutes or an hour, or however long you have energy and are having fun. Time can really fly when playing this game.

Also, this game can be played with anyone, not just someone you're in a relationship with. It could be a friend, family member, carer and doesn't have to be in pairs. There are so many ways to connect, to touch and be touched, which this game can help you discover.

One of the first (out of possibly hundreds) times I played this, I wasn't sure what to ask for. So, of course, I asked for a shoulder massage. Then, that became a slow back scratch. Then full body soft touch and I was amazed at how starting simply and being left wanting more (thanks to that timer) guided me to what I would like next. Asking for what you want can be difficult at first, but this game allows you to develop that skill with practice. Asking for what we want is such an essential skill to have during cancer treatments (and always).

A common question when introducing the two-minute game in workshops is, "what happens if someone asks for something you don't want to do?" Say "no-thank you" with a smile and discuss an alternative (such as touching the chest or back rather than genitals). It's okay. Wait, it's more than okay, it's wonderful to say 'no'. Saying what we don't want is equally (maybe more) important than saying what we do want. The goal is to find that optimal place where everyone is happy giving and receiving.

Here's a few reasons why this game can work for you:
Our genitals aren't always up for being played with, so when it's your two minutes, ask for something that doesn't include them (you have your whole body).

This game can allow connection, even with different levels of energy, libido, or when penetrative sex is not possible. Someone might want sexual touch for two minutes and if you're happy to give it, great! Your two minutes could be something that suits your mood such as "tell me your favourite joke using your hand as a puppet". The possibilities are endless and you can ask for exactly what you want, while easily avoiding what you don't want.

Bodies impacted by treatment can change dramatically and unpredictably, be it sensation, arousal, pain, surgical sites etc. This game allows you to relearn how your body works or doesn't work (where those desensitised parts are, where it's sore, where it's pleasurable, how toys or lubes feel).

If you're playing this with a partner and are worried about where things may lead to? Take 'typical' sex off the table for the entire game. You could have a 'no genital contact' rule or even leave your clothes on. Remove the pressure to perform or get aroused. Obligation & expectation are the enemy of arousal, feeling safe and relaxed is its catalyst. Get creative, enjoy yourselves without that pressure. You can enjoy pleasure from soft intimate touch anywhere on the body.

The two-minute game has many communication benefits and can act as a gentle ice breaker. With changed sexuality and changed intimacy (with or without illness), can come distance and avoidance. Talking about sex is not easy, especially when things are different. This game gently offers a way to help navigate those tricky feelings while also acknowledging the elephant in the room. While we're at it, let's erase any feelings of 'being selfish' or 'a taker'. Asking for your neck to be gently kissed for two minutes, or to be told why this person loves you for two minutes, is simply playing the game. It can seem difficult, but remember, you have to ask, it's the rules! Through my work as a sexuality and consent workshop facilitator, I'm always shocked at how many people tell me that they have never asked for what they want before. Practice makes perfect and it does get easier the more you do it.

Here's a list of things you could ask for, for your two minutes:

- Can you please lower the lights, put some relaxing music on that I would like, bring me water and join me on the couch in two minutes?

- Hold my hand and tell me how you're doing for two minutes.

- Massage my (insert body part here) for two minutes.

- Starting at my neck, ever so softly touch my entire

body, back to feet over two minutes.

- Tell me about your day through interpretive dance.

- Put on a song and show me your silliest/favourite dance move.

- Make me a cup of tea in two minutes.

- I would like to cuddle for two minutes.

- I would like to offer you a shoulder massage for two minutes (that's still your two minutes, but if you're not up for being touched, you can touch others. It's all about what YOU want).

- Massage my head.

- I would like to stroke your hair with your head in my lap.

- Lightly touch my beautiful bald head for 2 minutes.

- Gently kiss my neck/chest/thighs/back for two minutes.

- Show me how you like to be kissed, for two minutes.

- Kiss my face and tell me things you love about me for two minutes.

- Softly breathe on my entire body, ending with my genitals for two minutes (YUM!).

If you're thinking, "ugh, whatever Tess. Some of us don't know how to just simply know what you want and ask for it." You're right, I hear you. None of us are taught this, but I have a solution for you. A beautiful baby-step towards the 2-minute game and flexing those 'asking' muscles, is by playing the previous activity 'chatty massage'.

Active receiving

'Active receiving' is a way to connect with a lover/partner to the level that is right for you, when you're not feeling sexy or like having sex, and maybe need a little bit more time to get those feelings flowing.

It's a one-way touch experience, and a great way to enjoy touch. I'll explain a little more. There are many expectations and misconceptions in intimate activities, and a super common one is that it should always be a two-way experience. You give and receive pleasure at the same time. Well, this doesn't necessarily always have to be the case, and I offer you a wonderful way to connect in a one-way touch format, very similar to 'chatty massage' mentioned previously. This is wonderful for people with mismatched libido, delayed arousal responses (detailed in the 'reactive versus proactive arousal' section), if someone is not wanting to receive intimate touch or may not know what they want at that moment, but would love to see a partner have pleasure and enjoy themselves.

How it works.

Someone lies/sits down (or is in any comfortable position), asks for what type of touch they want, and constantly directs that person in how they touch them. The other person does exactly what they are being told to do. That's it! It's incredibly fun and accessible.

Imagine the person giving the touch and receiving the directions has no mind of their own, they are an inanimate object that only responds to commands. For the person following instructions, it can free you from that common brain chatter ("am I doing this right? Are they enjoying this? Are they pretending?"), as you're just doing what you're told.

Some examples of directions the person who is receiving touch (and giving all directions) could give are: "Massage my shoulders. Can you now scratch my back? Yum, thanks, can you go slower and a bit firmer? Softly touch my body up and down, neck to feet with your fingertips and don't stop until I say. Now, lightly pinch my inner thighs. Breathe cool breath on my nipples." Anything you want, just ask.

Unlike in chatty massage where the person following directions stops all together if they don't hear anything after a short while, in 'Active Receiving', the person giving the touch can check in to see if it's how the receiver wants it ("How is this pressure? Would you like me to move my hands faster or slower?") *without* stopping. The person following directions doesn't change anything, doesn't alter any style without being directed. If the person giving touch doesn't receive any directions for a while and isn't sure if this is still what the person receiving still wants? Keep doing what you were last asked to do and ask the question "how could you enjoy this more?"

Similar to chatty massage, this is an incredible skill to learn in the bedroom. Giving directions, asking for what we want, checking in with a lover to get feedback on their level of enjoyment, communicating your desires, all of this leads to better communication and better sex. If you get tired? Simply stop the activity whenever one of you wants. The goal is to enjoy receiving and to enjoy giving. 1 minute, 10 minutes, 20 minutes, it's all perfect.

If you're unsure, give it a go, clothes on, on the couch,

using just an arm or hand. Practice following directions, practice giving directions, practice checking in and identifying what you want. There is no goal here, just to have a touch experience, to give or receive pleasure, and enjoy connecting with a partner. It may feel clunky at first, but with practice it flows very easily and you will be amazed at how much you learn about your partner and their body (and yours!).

If this sounds like fun to you, but asking for what you want and giving directions seems a bit daunting, or taking directions and not being the one driving the experience sounds tough, I recommend playing 'chatty massage' or the '2-minute game' a few times first, before jumping into this activity. I say this only because it won't be enjoyable if you're still getting used to these styles of intimate communication. Those two activities are a wonderful (and fun!) way to develop these amazing sexy skills.

6. LUBE IS LIFE (& OTHER SAFETY ITEMS)

I want to march the streets of every major city across the globe, with thousands of chanting companions screaming for the use of lube. Lubricants are one of the most important and most underused sexual aids. Lube is your lovely friend, the friend that is easily and readily available any time you need it. It makes you feel comfortable and safe, and helps you feel good.

Remember, lubricants don't heal pain, they prevent it. But when you're at a point where your pain has lessened and you're willing to explore internal play again, finding the right one can make the world of difference for your comfort, and also future pain prevention. This section is for just that, to help you know your options and find what's best for you.

Some people say, "But I've never had to use lubricant before. It's never been *needed*," or, "I get my partner/s aroused enough, thanks". Lubricant isn't about mimicking or replacing arousal, it doesn't mean you're doing something wrong; it means you're doing something right.

Regardless of your age or your body, lubricant can enhance sexual activity, make it feel better, help it last longer and help make it safer. If sex is toast, lube is the spread. It's a bit like how food tastes good, but add a bit of salt or seasoning and suddenly it's so much better. Some of you might be thinking, "I've always used lube, it's awesome." That's great, keep going!

So, what are they, really? Lubricants are a viscous (slippery) liquid used to reduce friction when two surfaces rub against each other. If you rub your two hands together, fast, right now, you'll hear the sound of the skin rubbing and your hands will get warm (friction does that). Now, put some lube on your hands, maybe some soap and water and rub your hands together again...it's smoother and nicer, isn't it? That's what lubes do, make two surfaces slippery. Lubricants increase comfort, pleasure and safety, as it protects your delicate genital and anal tissues. What's more important than our safety?

Safety can mean many things. For anuses, penises or vaginas that are dry or sore, lubricants create extra moisture to relieve friction and *enhance* sensation. It protects barriers like condoms and dams, and most importantly, the moisture helps protect the skin from tearing. Skin tears can be uncomfortable, painful, decrease pleasure and also increase infection risk. Lubricants also reduce the risk of condoms breaking (whether on an object or genitals) as a dry environment can pull/rub on the barrier and strain it, or even tear it. Lubricants contribute to a safer sexual experience, and allow you to relax and enjoy more. If you're using lubricants and you're still feeling discomfort, please speak with your treating team.

If it goes in, put it on

The simple rule with lube is this: If anything is going to be inserted anywhere? Make sure it's clean, covered, and use lube. This includes tampons if you're feeling sore, tight or dry. Lube is nothing to be ashamed of or embarrassed about. Have it on your bedside table loud and proud, it shows you care about your and your lovers' well-being.

In Australia you can buy lubricants at your supermarket, local chemist, corner store and petrol station. If you don't want to buy lubricant in person, not a problem. They are easily purchased online and you can order small tubes/small amounts when you're first finding what you like, to avoid breaking the budget. Plus, online stores have more variety and much better quality than what you generally find in your local shop. Lubricants aren't expensive, so you can try many types to work out which ones you like as it makes a big difference to get a lubricant that suits you.

You can get everything from really basic to super organic to extremely fancy. It's about finding what suits you best, but I'll say this. Lubricants are like aeroplane tickets; you get what you pay for. It can be worth spending a little more for a better experience, especially if you have sensitive skin or atrophy, as the cheaper items may have more chemicals in them and cause a reaction.

What's out there?

There's quite a few different types of lubricants and moisturisers, and it can seem a bit daunting. Don't worry, I've broken it down, so you can find what's good for you.

<u>Water-based:</u>

In Australia you can get these everywhere, and are usable on toys and latex condoms. Water-based lubricants are easily absorbed by our bodies, so it's normal if you need to keep applying. Plus, if you like it very runny, you can also add more water to a water-based lube. Please don't think there is anything wrong if you need to keep adding more during play, it simply means your body is doing what it's designed to do, absorb water. When it comes to water-based lubricants, more is more.

Silicone based:

These lubricants are perfectly safe and are longer lasting, so you don't have to reapply as often as water-based lubes, plus they feel wonderful. Something most silicone lubes are not good for is to use them with silicone toys as it can damage the toy over time. If you're not sure, go to the website of the particular brand you're interested in to see if they specify it's safe to use on a silicone toy or not. Generally found in the FAQ section if their website has one. Toys made of other materials such as stainless steel, rubber, vinyl or glass are fine with this type of lube. If you want to use a silicone toy with your silicone lube, simply pop a condom over the toy creating a barrier between the two. If choosing is a bit overwhelming, I use Überlube and Sliquid Silver, they're so great.

Hybrid:

This means water-based mixed with silicone, it's a 'hybrid'

of the two main types of lubricants out there. These lubes last longer than solely water-based lubes as they're mixed, however they still do get absorbed by the body over time, as there is high water content.

Oil-based:

Oil based lubricants such as organic coconut oil or organic castor oil and more, are used by some and certainly work as a lubricant skin-to-skin, however there are a few things to mention. Oil-based lubricants can break down some latex materials which means that it's best to avoid oil-based lubricants when barriers (like latex condoms) are being used. You can buy condoms that are made out of other materials than latex, which are fine with oil-based products. Also, for those who have a vagina, oil-based lubricants can be thicker and harder for the internal tissues to flush out. I know many people who use organic coconut oil as a lubricant (and is great for massage oil), but have caution as it can cause thrush in some. A way to test this is to put a dab of oil on your inner thigh/outer labia to look for any reactions first.

Wax-based:

I'm referring to a particular product here because wax-based lubes aren't a huge thing (yet), but a pelvic floor physiotherapist in Australia created an 'intimate cream' made from beeswax and olive oil called 'olive & bee'. As described in the vaginal atrophy section, it can be used as a lubricant and also as an internal moisturiser. I have a few favourite lubes and moisturisers I like to use and this is in my top three. I use it as both a lubricant and a moisturiser. The beeswax is thick and creates a protective barrier, the olive oil has healing properties and because it's so thick and slick, it's pretty great for people with vulva & vaginal atrophy (hence why I love it so much). If you're UTI or thrush prone, have caution as this is a thick product and may be difficult for your vagina to flush out any remnants. A sterile lubricant may suit you better.

Sterile lubricants:

Generally, water-based, sterile lubes are commonly used in hospitals and clinical settings. It's as the name sounds, sterile. With a lower infection risk, this lube is used by medical professionals and is excellent to use with toys, especially toys/items that will penetrate. Remember me mentioning our very delicate internal tissues? Sterile lubricants can offer that extra layer of safety in case of any tissue damage. They are easily purchased online from medical stores and some online sex stores also. Plus, if you're UTI prone, sterile lubricants can be great as they have such a lower infection risk.

Chemicals:

Avoiding lubricants with high chemical content is recommended. So, don't purchase lubes that are coloured, scented or flavoured. Also, check the ingredient listing on the product label for parabens or other chemically sounding things, as they can irritate the skin. Essentially, if you're reading the ingredients list and you see a word so long you want to buy a vowel in order to be able to read it…..I'd give that word a good old google before buying the product. There are also 100% natural organic options which are easily found online. I've recently discovered lubricants containing colloidal silver, which has anti-inflammatory properties, can reduce itching and burning, promotes healing and doesn't disturb the oh-so-important natural pH levels inside us. This is a very gentle product, so again, if you're someone with discomfort or dryness, this could be a great one to try.

Lubricants used for anal-play:

For anal penetration, it's recommended by many in the industry to use thicker, more viscous lubricants (avoid lubricants with glycerin as they can get sticky and create friction). As a very important job of the rectum is to absorb water, silicone-based lubricants can be great for the anus as there is less water in them, so they last longer. There are also water-based lubricants which are thicker and specially designed for anal play, these are also great, but you *must* make sure they specify they are for anal use.

Remember, a standard water-based lubricant will be absorbed quickly into your body and you may experience friction if you don't top up regularly. Whether you're on treatments or not, lubricants are essential as our anuses don't produce moisture on their own, so lubricant makes everything more comfortable. The tissues are quite delicate in there, so if you warm-up your anus (a bit of foreplay doesn't hurt anyone - literally!) and use lubricants, you will avoid causing any damage. As I keep saying, the anus is a highly pleasurable area of the human body and it needs care before being played with.

Vaginal moisturisers:

As discussed previously in the 'our poor vajootz' section, internal moisturisers are exactly what they sound like. A moisturiser that gets applied internally inside the vagina, repeatedly over a period of time. Some are only accessible via a script from your oncologist which may contain hormones, others such as 'intrarosa' mimic the steroid 'prasterone' and others are available at pharmacies on the shelf. Please ask your doctor before purchasing one and speak with the pharmacist when you're there, about the medications you're on. There may be ingredients that will cause a reaction to your internal tissues, the only way to know if something could benefit you, is to consult with your treating team.

Some vaginal moisturisers have hormones such as oestrogen in them, so if your cancer is hormone receptive, this may have negative impacts. It may be fine, but better to be sure and safe. You will need to speak to your oncologist to ask if a vaginal moisturiser is appropriate for you to use and they will recommend what is best for you. There are hormone free moisturisers on the chemist and pharmacy shelves, some need prescriptions from doctors, and others you can order online. If you need a hormone free internal moisturiser, look for anything that contains hyaluronic acid. It's a slick substance we produce naturally in our bodies to keep our synovial joints moving smoothly and it's great for our internal tissues.

There are also moisturisers which can be used externally, for the vulva area. Again, you will need to consult your treating team to see what is recommended as having the right cream is vital to avoid potential harm. This is one of those times where you really must ask.

Using lube with barriers

Lubricants need to be put on after the safer sex barrier is in place. If lube is put on the body part or toy before the barrier, you're creating a slippery surface under the barrier and there is a much greater risk (almost a guarantee) of it coming/sliding off during play.

- If you're using a condom for a penis or toy to be inserted into something, put the condom on first, then the lube on the condom covered penis/toy.

- If you're using an internal condom for a vagina or anus, put the condom inside the person first, then the lube. Also, with internal condoms, the lube can also go on the thing that will penetrate, such as a toy, finger or penis before insertion.

- If you're using a condom for an individual finger, pop the condom over the finger, then put lube over the condom-covered finger.

- Regardless of treatment, if you're going to insert anything, anywhere, put a condom on it and then lube on the condom. This is an extra way to ensure cleanliness and hygiene and also makes cleaning the toy/object/person much easier.

Gloves

Gloves are a wonderful and versatile safer sex item. If you're touching someone's genitals and feel you have dirt under your fingernails or perhaps some cuts and abrasions on your hand/fingers, pop some gloves on. Most importantly, is to mention that gloves don't remove all sensory feedback, as the person wearing gloves, you can still feel plenty.

Gloves also feel excellent on skin, for the person being touched. They're just another way to explore and enjoy new and different sensory experiences. There are several types of gloves, vinyl, latex or Nitrile. Nitrile gloves are easily accessed online, feel pretty great and are perfect for the people out there who have latex allergies.

7. A QUICK NOTE ON HYGIENE

Self-care regimes during treatments can be exhausting, however it's very important to stay clean to lower infection risk and prevent discomfort. I'm not saying that you need to shower three times a day, but at least once a day is necessary. It's important to keep your body clean and refreshed, but remember, our genitals need particular care as they have such soft and sensitive tissues, and treatments can make our genitals more sensitive and irritated. So, we want them to be clean, but we also don't want to irritate them further with soaps that can wash away all of the protective and amazing natural bacteria we have around and inside our genitals. Too much washing (especially with soaps) can actually cause more irritation, so here's some tips.

- Wipe front to back after going to the toilet to prevent thrush and UTIs. If you're sore externally, gently dab yourself dry with paper.
- Wash your genitals with warm (not hot) water. Avoid using things like a flannel or sponge, as they can scratch and irritate the skin.

- As with lubricants, also avoid perfumed soaps or soaps that have chemicals. Warm water is usually sufficient, but if you want to use soap, make sure it's pH balanced and specify on the label that it's for 'intimate areas'. This applies for all genital configurations. These soaps are available on the shelf in Australian chemists and supermarkets (and online anywhere in the world).

- The vagina has a self-cleaning system, which is why we so often have discharge in our underwear. If you notice a change in smell, please don't use soaps internally (never use soaps internally!), continue to wash externally with warm water and let your vagina clean itself out as it's designed to do. If things don't seem quite right, chat with your doctor.

- When you're drying yourself after a shower or bath, gently pat your genitals dry with your clean towel. You want to avoid rubbing and scraping type motions.

- Avoid perfumes and deodorants in those areas and looser fitting clothing can help the skin breathe if you're feeling sensitive.

- If you use pantyliners, change them regularly and only use them when needed. They're not for everyday use as they trap in warmth and moisture. Period underwear breathe and are great if you change them each morning and night.

8.   UH-OH, WHERE'S MY O?
(CHANGES IN ORGASM)

Something not often spoken about is how during and after cancer treatments your orgasms/climax can change, or sometimes even disappear.

It's essential we do not have penetrative sex while it hurts, however once the pain has eased and this type of sex is possible once more, people sometimes have trouble reaching orgasm or they feel different once they resume penetrative forms of sex. This is common (it happened to me and many others I support), this is normal, you are normal.

How can they change, you ask? Maybe they're less 'intense', maybe they're more intense. Perhaps you need a lot more time and play (yum!) to 'get there', maybe your body shakes and does the things it normally does, but you don't really feel any actual orgasm. What I call a *'ghost-gasm'*, and was very strange to me during chemo when I first experienced this. There is also the possibility that orgasms and climaxes may not be possible for a while. Sex can still be very pleasurable during cancer treatments, but sometimes our medications or nervousness block that 'peak-climactic' experience.

Thanks to the wonders of neuroscience, we now know that our body can 100% relearn how to have them, or have *different* ones.

If you would like to relearn how to have orgasms, or better put, if you would like to rewire your pleasure so the body you now have can have climaxes (even if they're a little different) here's something to try.

Regular self-pleasure with a few rules
I'm talking even just 2-5 minutes a day (10 would be better).

1. Remove the goal, remove the pressure
Ban the orgasm. You heard me! You're only allowed to touch and enjoy your body to rewire your brain and associate touch with *'goal-free'* pleasure. This neurologically starts to rewire your brain in the background that intimacy isn't about the pressure of that goal. This creates freedom and can be a major stepping stone to your pleasure and orgasm recovery. Better yet, if you have a partner/s, have a 'no orgasm allowed' touch-fest a few times a week. Even if you currently can't orgasm, removing it verbally anyway

allows you to enjoy the touch you're receiving (without the guilt, pressure and frustration). Remember, removing the goal can help you get to the goal. You can do this with a partner, but if so, put a timer on and you're only allowed to touch while the timer (5-10mins) is on. It's another way to remove that expectation of it having to 'go somewhere' or 'achieve something'.

2. Don't forget to breathe.

Breath is powerful, as it not only can be used to down or up-regulate our nervous system, but it also aids in circulating blood to our internal tissues. So many of us tense up and hold our breath when we're in pleasure or when we're *trying* to have an intense moment. It's like we're forcing an orgasm to arrive, which is going to get in the way of you having one! It's like trying to force yourself to go to sleep, the effort of forcing it counteracts where you want to go.

Next time you're having pleasure (with yourself or another), relax your muscles and slow down your breath. Remember, this is about pleasure not orgasms, so be curious. Relaxing your body and making sure you're breathing gets blood flow to the deep internal tissues. With blood flow, the tissues get oxygenated and guess what? Our sensitivity increases and so does our pleasure!

If you notice you're tense and/or hold your breath in pleasure, have a few practice runs with yourself. Touch your body, experience pleasure and arousal, but when you notice your muscles tensing up or you're holding your breath, stop, slow down, and only continue when you're relaxed again. Think of it like a pleasure meditation. It can feel strange, but trust me, blood-flow is the key to arousal and pleasure, and we can't circulate blood without breath, and blood can't reach our internal pleasure structures without those muscles being relaxed.

3. Slow it down.

Some of my work includes masturbation coaching with clients, teaching people that there's more than just fast-paced/standard movements. When we rush, we get distracted and then that '*should*' brain (the obligation and pressure of getting somewhere) can get in the way. Plus, as just mentioned, going slow allows blood circulation and muscles to relax... again, blood-flow increases our sensation, arousal and our pleasure. Cancer treatments often give us a slower arousal response, so we need more time to really get into it. Orgasms may be achievable; they just need more time and 'warm-up'. If this is you, take a look at the 'toys' section a little later, I have some suggestions for you.

4. Massage

A number one way to recover orgasm is through genital massage (refer to the 'Vulva Pleasure Masterclass' in the 'resources' section at the end). We all love massage, it's relaxing, allows our muscles to relax and can reduce tightness while increasing blood-flow. Vulvovaginal massage is incredible for orgasm recovery on many levels. Through various massage techniques you can recover and discover new pleasure zones and enhance sensitivity.

5. Repetition.

To make change neurologically you need time and repetition. Self-pleasure and/or massage regularly. A few times a week, over months, maybe 5 mins of loving touch every day if you can (but a few times a week if that's more doable for you). Pleasure rewiring is not a quick fix, but from someone who's been-there-done-that after treatments, it can be done!

6. Exercise.

I've discussed this already so will be super brief here, but exercise helps with arousal as it gets blood-flow to the deeper pelvis structures, engorging tissues and heightening sensitivity. If you can find even just 10 minutes to go for a quick walk or jog, or do some yoga before a pleasure session, this can help increase your sensitivity and arousal, helping pave the way towards orgasms.

7. Lastly, TOYS.

Explore with vibration as it offers stimulation to the deeper tissues and in a way we can't offer naturally. It's a great kick-starter for those times when you want to experience pleasure, but aren't sure exactly what your body enjoys. If you're not sure where to start looking (as the range of intimacy toys is endless), refer to the upcoming section titled 'it's toy time'.

Firstly, the vagina is not designed to have peak orgasmic experiences, the clitoris is. And although most of our clitoral structure is inside us, we do have a portion of it externally/on the outside of our body for easy access. So, you could try stimulating the head of your clitoris (the part of the clitoris you can touch on the outside of your body) before and during play as a way to warm-up and kick-start your reactive arousal.

Finally, please know there is nothing wrong with using toys. Just like we use glasses to read better, we can use toys to pleasure better. And toy shopping with a partner? Best foreplay ever!

A quick note, that there are some countries which legally sell THC and cannabis products and some folks tell me that specific strains can influence arousal and their ability to climax. I cannot make recommendations as unfortunately Australia is a little behind and it's not legal here, so I can't access this product. I feel it would be irresponsible of me not to mention this, for those who live in countries and specific states of the US that can access this, and may want to look into it further.

This is very general advice and I know our bodies are much more complicated than a few simple steps, but the information here is truly powerful. Our desire and arousal are so complicated during and after cancer treatments, and also for partners. Be kind to yourselves, this is tough and the changes in your body may well be temporary.

9. IT'S TOY TIME!

In this section, I'm going to be discussing a few toys out there. I'll never be able to cover it all as it's endless. So, I'm only going to be chatting about a few *types* of toys that I often recommend to clients, who are experiencing changes in their arousal and pleasure.

Firstly, and most importantly. Toys don't mean something is wrong, toys mean something is right! Think of it, the word 'toy' is perfect. It's about fun, it's about play. Approaching sex with playfulness, exploration and curiosity is how to ensure you have a good time on so many levels.

I'm going to start with vibration, as it's a wonderful tool to use for people that have mismatched libido and delayed arousal, or sore tissues that could use a bit of healing internally. They can also be a very useful (and fun) way to get someone into their pleasure quicker.

Vibration

Toys that vibrate have a few main purposes which are to offer heightened stimulation and to access deeper tissues. There are countless types of vibration toys and I'll cover a few, but remember this. Vibration is a wonderful method to offer a type of stimulation to parts of our body that we can no longer stimulate ourselves and also offers stimulation in a way we cannot do naturally or anymore. Plus, vibration is felt *deeper* in the body, so it can be more arousing because it reaches more tissues internally. If we're experiencing numbness or changes in sensation and pleasure, exploring with vibration can be a way to stimulate our arousal, when things aren't working the same as they used to.

There are vibrators for penises, vaginas, anuses, the clitoris and there are so many to choose from.

They can be used at the beginning of play, to kind of kick-start pleasure and arousal. They can be used during play, to maintain arousal or increase pleasure. They can be used at the end of play, if perhaps someone wants to heighten their pleasure in the hopes of reaching climax with another partner, or to 'finish-off'.

Or all of the above.

They're also great for vaginal atrophy, that dry sandpaper feeling internally during penetrative sex, as vibrations applied externally on your body (say on the head of your clitoris) stimulates blood flow to the area. Vibration can also be great for people that have changes in genital sensation and may be experiencing 'numbness' and can be a great way to 'wake up' the sensory receptors.

There is no right or wrong way to use them, as long as you're exploring and going slowly the first few times you play with them. When our bodies change, so does our sensitivity, so we can 'overload' ourselves if we go too fast too soon.

I'm going to now introduce you to a very popular vibration toy called the 'doxy wand'.

Doxy massager wand:
The original model was a 'Hitachi wand', which is almost identical to the 'doxy wand', known to be one the most intense vibration toys that exist and were originally designed for deep tissue massage. There are many models available including less expensive ones with a slightly less powerful motor (I think if you type in Amazon or eBay 'body massager' you'll find a bunch). These toys are not designed for internal use, but the vibration is so strong you

feel it throughout your whole body regardless.

This toy is wonderful when being held against a vulva, clitoris, anus and that magical perineal space between the scrotum and anus or between the vagina and anus.

You *must* start slowly, at the lowest setting. If you start at a higher setting, you may get overwhelmed. This is also wonderful for massage and if you're getting intimate with a partner and offering sensual touch, pop this out and use it for relaxation. It's amazing on the lower back and shoulders and helps me get through migraines when I use it on my neck.

Tip #1; When you're using it, pop a condom over the head and a few drops of lube. That way when you're done you can simply pull the condom off and give it a wash in soapy warm water and it's perfectly clean. Plus, with the lube it just makes things smoother and more enjoyable (we always want to prevent friction).

Tip #2; You can use this toy through your hand by placing it on the back of your hand while you're touching someone. This is the toy that can magically turn your hand or fingers into a vibrating hand! And yes, it most definitely does feel good (a friend of a friend told me).

Clitoral vibrators:

Another amazing vibratory toy which also uses air-pulses is a clitoral vibrator.

These toys vibrate and gently suck and pulse air. Anyone using this *must* start at the lowest setting and go slowly, as you want to find what's right for your body. This can be used on a clitoris, the head of a penis (soft or hard) or the nipples. Again, use a few drops of lubricant on the area you're pleasuring.

You can find these toys (there's a few brands) online by searching the word 'clitoris' or 'clitoral vibrator' and they'll come up.

As mentioned, these toys are great for getting blood-flow to promote healing to your vaginal tissues without having to be penetrated, for mismatched libido and for anyone and everyone with delayed/reactive arousal. They feel absolutely *sensational* and are small enough to be used during play alone or with (or by) another. This is a really handy toy to have when someone may need a little more time and pleasure to get aroused. Just be curious, go slow and get to know it. I'm yet to recommend this toy to someone and have them report back to me as anything but happy.

Anal toys

Anal pleasure has quite a bad reputation, but is a sexual part of our body that is capable of soooooo much pleasure! And is a wonderful way to have amazing peak-pleasure experiences when our vaginas are offline. Want to know the number one way to experience anal pleasure? GO SLOW! The slower, the better, as when our mind is tense, or we're feeling nervous, we clench our muscles and sphincters, which gets in the way of it feeling good. Relaxation is everything and wow, can this be an amazing way to have pleasure! I've helped people who could no longer orgasm and be penetrated vaginally gently explore this part of their body, and wow, were they blown away!

There are so many varieties of anal toys and I could speak on the topic of anal pleasure forever (and do when I'm running anal-pleasure workshops), so I'm going to keep this super basic.

Most people have had a bad anal experience in sex, for various reasons and most people I coach feel that because they didn't enjoy it then, means they don't enjoy it at all.

The anus is designed and capable of extreme pleasure, but needs to be relaxed to be ready (like the rest of our body) for play and penetration. Start with gentle massage, hold some vibration on the outside of the sphincter (like using the doxy wand resting against your finger, so your vibrating fingertip is stimulating the anal entrance), breathe and give your body and mind time to relax.

Always start with the smallest toys. Buy the smallest butt-plug and only put the tip in, get used to the sensations. In the shower when you're washing, give the outside of your anus a few moments of soft curious touch.

Vibrating butt-plugs are *amazing* and are great for getting blood to that area. Always start small, start slow, start with curiosity. Bigger is not better, what's good for you is what's best for you.

The blindfold

Yes, this is a sex toy, as well as an object of daily function. This simple and easily found item is a real game changer.

The blindfold can really help quiet that brain-chatter by removing visible distractions and is great to help calm our mind when we're anxious or self-conscious. Plus, when we remove one of our senses, all of the others get heightened.

Touch just gets better with a blindfold on. Through decreasing distraction and increasing your sensitivity, this can be a great way to find those erogenous and pleasure zones you never thought existed for greater pleasure. I highly recommend.

Things to consider when buying a toy

<u>Shape</u>. Can you hold it? Is it a shape you could use in your hands (too small, too thin, too large, too wide)?

<u>Buttons</u>. Are the buttons on it large enough for you to use? If you have arthritis or peripheral neuropathy, you may want to choose a toy where the buttons are on the larger side.

<u>Sound</u>. Does it use a motor and if so, does it mention intensity of sound? I often look for toy descriptors that mention things like 'whisper quiet'. If you live in a tiny apartment like I do, I have to consider my neighbours. I always look for 'quieter' toys.

<u>Collaborative</u>. Could a partner or date use the toy on you also? Not a necessity, but does mix things up and creates

other levels of fun!

Solo. Can you use this toy on yourself? If you're a bit nervous and new to intimacy aids, going slow and trying it gently on yourself a few times alone can be wonderful if you want to enjoy it with others.

Disability. If you have impaired upper limb function, does this toy come in a box with lots of packaging, have small tiny cable inserts to charge, does it need to be taken apart and put back together again to be cleaned, or is it functional only through pushing small buttons? There aren't many intimacy aids out there for people with limited hand function, so I want to specifically mention the 'Bump'n joystick' and 'the Ziggy' by LUDDI. These toys were both designed by people with disability and healthcare clinicians, specifically for folks with impacted upper limb and hand movement (see the 'resources' section for more info). They're amazing.

So, we've covered some basics in what is an endless topic. Remember, toys are exactly that, toys. They are fun! But also have a lot of benefits post cancer diagnosis as mentioned previously.

If you're not sure where to start, google 'online sex toy store (and your city/country name)'. You will find some.

Check posting to your country, read the reviews online and if they have it available, watch any short videos on how to use the toy. The international online toy store 'Lovehoney' has lots of 1–2-minute videos on their toys, if you're interested to shop and learn. This can seem a little daunting, but just like everything else in sexuality, approach it with curiosity and exploration, you'll be fine.

10. TIPS FOR LOVED ONES

Communicating with your partners

Pop-quiz, what am I?

We're not supposed to talk about it, you can't have too much of it, you can't have too little of it, it's used in nearly all marketing to sell but it's never presented accurately in the media, it's a part of human life, social media platforms shut you down for talking about it, people who are different, unwell, older, living with disability, are of different cultures and ethnicities are assumed to not have it or to want it, we receive no education on it yet we're supposed to magically be good at it and we're supposed to always want it....... Yup. That'd be sex.

You may feel from reading the above that you can't win, and sure, our culture doesn't exactly embrace open communication regarding sexuality, but reading this book is how you will learn.

In my experience as a sexuality educator (as well as from my own life), people who are able to talk between themselves about sex more openly, have much better sex. Why, you ask? Because communicating about how you're feeling and what you might enjoy, allows you to engage comfortably and pleasurably. It can also reduce feeling like you're forcing yourself, forcing someone else, or causing any possible harm. It's okay if things have changed, our bodies and pleasure always will. If we can learn how to communicate about what we do or don't want, things will be better. Remember, hand holding, eye contact, cuddles, snuggles on the couch, foot/body/hand massage, genital massage, oral genital play, assisting/giving masturbation, self-touch together, watching pornography together or reading erotic literature together, all of these things are sex and all of them are connective.

Seeing a loved one go through cancer is tough, and so can knowing what to say or how to act. Whether you're a carer, friend, family member or partner, there are ways to offer connection without overstepping a line. And don't worry, we won't break!

Yes, caution is (very) necessary and the medical team must tell you about all of the risks involved in all treatments. People undergoing chemo, surgeries, radiotherapy, we can be seen as easily hurt, fragile or dangerous, and rightly so. There are many side-effects of treatments, some of them are mental and some of them are physical. However, let's remember this: connection is always important, and even if someone's body and mind are changing, there are still ways to be there with someone.

I dive into the impacts of particular treatments soon; however, it can understandably be hard to know what to do. It's also normal, when seeing a loved one be so unwell, to want to avoid causing any other harm and through that, create physical distance. That might look like reducing touch and physical contact, or even like possible avoidance. If you're a partner, lover, friend or carer of someone during treatment, I implore you, I beg you, to offer them touch. Treatment is damaging and also detaching. We need the treatment, yes, but we also need care, to feel connected to ourselves and to those around us. Don't be afraid of us, be cautious and curious with us. Think of it as getting into 'ask first' mode.

For simple touch, a peck on the lips or cheek? It's okay! We are not radioactive, we won't give you cancer and we won't break, if we all just take a little care. How do we know what to do or what not to do? We ask.

How to say it out loud.

- "Would you like me to take your hand?"

- "Is there any way you might like some loving/comforting touch right now?"

- "Would you like a hug?"

- "I'd love a cuddle; how does that sound to you?"

- "I'd love to connect with you, are there any sore spots I should avoid if I went in for a cuddle?"

- "I'd love to connect with you right now, is there a form of touch you would like?" (Arm around the shoulder, hand holding, hug from behind, foot massage and more)

- "I love you and want to offer you affection, is there anything that would comfort you at the moment?"

- "I miss you, but I'm worried I'll hurt you if I squeeze you too hard. Is there a way I can snuggle into you?"

- "I'm wanting to show you love and affection, such as a kiss on the lips or cheek, how do you feel about that?"

- "I'm checking you out right now, fancy a kiss?"

If you're being made an offer of connection and it's not a good time? I offer some examples shortly on ways to navigate that, however a simple, "thank you, but I'm not quite up for it at the moment" is perfect. Even if the person receiving this offer is not up for it right then, you're showing love, care, concern for their well-being and the desire to remain connected. It means the world.

Not in the mood?

Whether you're the person with cancer or the partner of, there will be times when you don't feel like being intimate with others, that is fine, that is normal, that is understandable. There will also be times when you feel like connecting somehow, but aren't sure how. There are lots of places to start: Get in the bath and relax or wrap yourself in blankets with a hot-water bottle, maybe touch your body, snuggle a pet with your favourite film, ask the person you're with to intertwine your legs while you both sit on the couch or lean into their chest. During treatments, you're not going to want intimacy or touch all of the time, so feel free to let loved ones know how you're feeling and speak up in the moments it seems plausible. If you do receive an offer of intimacy and connection and you're not up for it? Remember, that's okay, that's fine, that's normal. But also remember to say thanks for the offer and be kind when you say no thanks, because you want the offers to keep coming!

How to say it out loud.

- "Thank you, that sounds amazing, it's not the best moment, can we see how I'm going later?" (Or tomorrow, or after lunch)

- "Thanks, I'm feeling quite nauseous/tired/in some pain, for the moment I need to sit still, can we maybe connect later or another day?"

- "I'm really not feeling well, I'd like to sit alone for a while. Thank you so much for offering a cuddle, rain-check?"

- "I'd love to kiss you, but my mouth is a bit sore at the moment, would you like some soft neck touch instead?"

- "I'd love a hug, thank you, could you be careful around my arm? It's a bit sore."

- "I don't think I'm up for a hug right now, would you like to hold my hand?"

- "I'm pretty low on energy at the moment, but something soft and gentle would be lovely, like a snuggle?"

- Or if you're ADHD and ridiculously blunt like me "Thanks for the offer of a kiss, I'm currently trying not to vomit in my mouth, so will need to rain-check" (we both had a giggle at that).

To those undergoing treatments, if you feel your partner/lover/friend is avoiding you, unattracted to you and doesn't want to touch you? They may just be thinking they are protecting you, avoiding potentially hurting you or feel like they're pestering/pressuring you, so are pulling away. Be the one to communicate and offer a connection. Offer to snuggle, offer to touch their back while they're standing next to you, ask for a long hug hello, it guides them, and can lead to further connections. It meant the world to me, having my hand held and legs entwined on the couch with a cup of tea and chats. It was meaningful and intimate, that at times was my sex. Simple things like that were so important, and I know is/was to others during treatments.

11. FOR MY FELLOW RAINBOW-FLAGGERS

For people in the LGBTQIA+ community, medical institutions can be very difficult. I remember sitting in the chemo-chair with my then partner holding my hand. The nurse approached and looked at us holding hands, then looking at her said "oh, isn't that sweet you're such good *friends*". I know the nurse meant well, but it was devaluing to me and my partner. I did not feel like I was seen as a person, nor my partner respected. I also did not have the energy to continually educate everyone around me all day every day and advocate for who I am and for others. It's exhausting and with cancer, I didn't have it in me. So, I withdrew and I became reluctant to share my personal story with most clinicians. This is particularly important for people with cancers such as prostate, testicular, cervix, ovaries or breast (just to name a few), as these cancers are *very* gendered. Due to this people can isolate themselves from the supports that are out there as they may feel unwelcome or unseen. Speaking personally, the 'sisterhood' is very strong in breast cancer and as a non-binary person, was difficult to ignore. I avoided so many (pretty much all) support networks due to this as I did not feel welcome. If you're someone who resonates with this, if you belong to communities that are marginalised, I ask you to reach out. Reach out to that one person on your treating team you can have an honest, non-shaming conversation with. Reach out to the nurse asking for any resources the hospital knows of that are accessible and inclusive. Reach out to a friend, to find a cancer support group near you or online that is gender aware, recognises pronouns, alternative relationship models, and partnerships that are not only heterosexual. They are out there, but you may need help finding them. Feeling safe and supported is everything.

RESOURCES

Because there's limited work on sexuality and cancer and well, actual realistic and accessible sexuality education in general, resources can be hard to find. So, here are some, of varied mediums depending on what suits you best.

The 'A Better Normal' mini-book series

Available globally on Amazon in paperback or eBook format, you can search by author 'Tess Devèze' or by book title.

If you're needing support, practical solutions and guidance on more specific side-effects, or looking for help regarding a specific treatment, the 'A Better Normal' mini-book series covers quite a range.

Books in the 'A Better Normal' mini-book series are:

- 'A Better Normal for **Libido**; Your Guide to Rediscovering Intimacy After Cancer'

- 'A Better Normal for **Vaginal Dryness & Pain**; Your Guide to Rediscovering Intimacy After Cancer'

- 'A Better Normal for **Body Confidence**; Your Guide to Rediscovering Intimacy After Cancer'

- 'A Better Normal for **Chemotherapy**; Your Guide to Rediscovering Intimacy After Cancer'
- 'A Better Normal for **Hormone Therapy**; Your Guide to Rediscovering Intimacy After Cancer'
- 'A Better Normal for **Fatigue**; Your Guide to Rediscovering Intimacy After Cancer'
- 'A Better Normal for **Changes in Erection**; Your Guide to Rediscovering Intimacy After Cancer'
- 'A Better Normal for **Radiotherapy**; Your Guide to Rediscovering Intimacy After Cancer'
- 'A Better Normal for **Pain**; Your Guide to Rediscovering Intimacy After Cancer'

The all-in-one resource, 'A Better Normal; Your Guide to Rediscovering Intimacy After Cancer'

Available globally on Amazon in paperback or eBook, you can search via author 'Tess Devèze' or by book title.

If you liked the information in this book, but feel you need guidance on more, the book 'A Better Normal; Your Guide to Rediscovering Intimacy After Cancer' has all of the information included in the entire mini-book series and more. It's your one stop shop for everything you need to know about sexuality and cancer, in the one book.

Vulva Pleasure Masterclass

(connectable.podia.com/vulva-masterclass)

For anyone with a vulva who is experiencing pain and dryness, or is experiencing loss of sensation, pleasure, arousal and orgasm. This online Masterclass teaches vulva massage, which can be done on yourself or with a partner. Through massage and neurological concepts, things like arousal and pleasure can be recovered while helping heal tissues through increasing blood-flow with massage. This Masterclass is also suitable for people with vaginismus and vulvodynia.

Penis Pleasure Masterclass

(connectable.podia.com/penis-pleasure)

For anyone with a penis who is experiencing changes in erection and orgasm, or is experiencing loss of sensation, function and pleasure. This online Masterclass teaches soft penis massage, which can be done on yourself or with a partner. Through massage and neurological concepts, things like sensation and pleasure can be recovered while helping recover erectile function through increasing blood-flow with massage. This Masterclass is particularly beneficial for people post prostatectomy.

A libido and intimacy recovery program for couples
'Connection & Cancer: Reclaim Your Intimacy & Desire'.
(connectable.podia.com/libido-after-cancer)

If you would like personal support through the exact process of *how* to recover your pleasure, intimacy and libido, then this is for you. It's with me online guiding you every step of the way, and is done in the privacy of your own home. Filled with information, fun and practical solutions that I take you through for libido recovery. The people who I've worked with in this program are having life-changing results. It's an absolute honour to guide people to recover what they felt was lost forever.

'ConnectAble Therapies' (connectabletherapies.com)
For consultations and further resources on sex, intimacy & cancer.

Facebook global support group: *'Intimacy and Cancer'.* This group is for any cancer, any gender and is a very supportive space.

Instagram '@connectable_therapies', where I regularly share helpful information.

YouTube Channel on sex, intimacy & cancer: type *"Intimacy and Cancer CHANNEL"* to find it.

If you prefer video formats over reading (as cancer-brain & reading don't go well together), this YouTube Channel is filled with short videos discussing all things sex, intimacy and cancer.

'ConnectAble Courses' (connectable.podia.com)

A site of intimacy and cancer online courses for sexual recovery. Including the Masterclasses, libido recovery program and webinar mentioned here.

Intimacy & Cancer Information Webinar

(connectable.podia.com/webinar-intimacyaftercancer)

A free information webinar discussing the impacts cancer treatments have on intimacy and sexuality. It has a particular focus on libido and how it can be recovered.

Other amazing resources:

'A Touchy Subject' (atouchysubject.com)

For people with prostate cancer or experiencing changes in erection. Victoria Cullen is *the* person to go to, about sexuality and intimacy post a prostate cancer diagnosis. She also has a YouTube channel and through her website access to free resources and rehabilitation programs.

'The Art of The Hook Up' (artofthehookup.com)
This site from dating expert and communication extraordinaire is by Georgie Wolf. Not cancer specific, but incredibly on-point and with relative information for anyone struggling with the dating scene. She has podcasts, blogs, eBooks and more. She's also a workshop facilitator and a bit of a superstar here in Australia!

'Curious Creatures' (curiouscreatures.biz)
For online workshops and much more education on self-development and sexuality. They provide articles, podcasts and streamable workshops which are all very practical and very accessible. I have the privilege to work for this company, their work is changing lives.

'Bump'n Joystick' (getbumpn.com)
An intimacy aid designed for people with impaired upper

limb and fine-motor function. Suitable for all genders and is flexible to varied body shapes. This toy was designed by the global disability and OT community, and it's pretty incredible.

'The Ziggy' (luddi.co)

Another intimacy aid designed for people with limited upper limb and intact fine-motor function. Designed by the disability community and healthcare professionals, this is a multi-purpose vibrator for all genders. It's also able to be used while in a wheelchair, so is a wonderfully accessible item.

Pelvic and sexual health osteopath

For those who live in Melbourne, Australia, we have one of the top pelvic health osteopaths you'll ever find. Dr Andrew Carr from the *'Whole Being Collective'* is referred to as *'the body whisperer'* in clinical and sexual health circles. He works with the entire body, however has expertise and clinical focus on pelvic and sexual health. In particular, people experiencing pelvic pain including after treatments, vaginismus, atrophy and is trauma informed.

If you're not located in Melbourne, there are pelvic

floor osteopaths, physiotherapists and OTs all over the world. Simply search online "Pelvic floor osteopath/physio/OT (insert the name of your city/town here)". You'll find someone near you.

Support groups in your area

If you search in google "Cancer Support (insert city/town where you live here)", there should be a list of businesses and companies that have programs near you. Some online or in person. They mightn't be sexuality specific, but there is always opportunity for discussions and learning.

ACKNOWLEDGEMENTS

For anyone and everyone out there affected by cancer, this book is for you. There can be so much to consider, to have to endure, to have to keep track of, that many parts of life take a back seat. Thank you for caring about your intimacy and connections during such a time, be it connections with yourself or with others. I hope you're supported and I truly hope there is something in this book for you.

I'm forever grateful to my clients and the thousands I support online who so openly and vulnerably share their struggles, and also their triumphs with me. This book would not exist without you. I'm inspired and amazed by you all, daily.

Thank you, to my partners and carers over the years Rog, Robi and Kane, my family and my global network of friends. There were some very dark places during treatments and you all got me through. To my booby buddies (my breast care nurses) Claire & Monique, you're my angels. Ricky Dick my oncologist - you're simply the best (Tina Turner style!) and to my RADelaidies.

Lastly, to acknowledge the incredible ethics, values and approaches to sexuality and communication from Roger

Butler at Curious Creatures (and their generosity with sharing their content with me), the occupational therapy & sexuality community (yeah OT-siggers!) and the revolutionary perspectives and therapeutic trainings I received from Deej & Uma, at the Institute of Somatic Sexology (ISS).

ABOUT THE AUTHOR

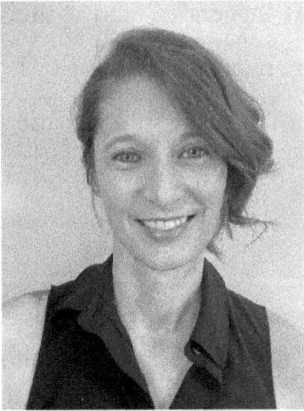

Tess Devèze is an occupational therapist (OT) having completed their bachelor degree in Melbourne Australia, founding ConnectAble Therapies, a community sexuality OT and sexology clinic focussing on sexuality and intimacy for people with neurological conditions, cancer, chronic illness and disability. They have also completed certification and trainings via the Institute of Somatic Sexology. Alongside being a sexuality OT, Tess is also a sexuality educator & workshop facilitator, and has facilitated and educated thousands of people in the topics of communication, consent, sexuality, pleasure and relationship dynamics for nearing a decade. Tess founded the global online initiative 'Intimacy and Cancer', an online support space for people of all cancers and genders to access sexual support.

As a non-binary, queer, disabled person living with cancer, Tess's work is inclusive and advocates for sexual rights for disabled, neurodivergent, gender queer/diverse and LGBTQIA+, communities, which they proudly belong to.

Tess was diagnosed with stage 3 breast cancer at the age of 36 and is still undergoing treatments.

Find them at www.connectabletherapies.com

DID YOU ENJOY THE BOOK?

As an independent author, my work survives through your support. There are so many people affected by cancer, suffering in silence. With each review or word-of-mouth recommendation you make, we can reach the many out there who are struggling and need support.

Please leave a review by visiting where you purchased this book. It's just 1 minute of your time, but could be the thing that helps this reach someone who needs it, someone who needs a better normal too.

Got feedback? Please leave a review! Plus, I'd love to hear from you. You can reach me via email at tess@connectabletherapies.com or via Instagram @connectable_therapies.